Nourish and Slim

A Guide to Diabetic Weight Loss Through Balanced Nutrition

TABLE OF CONTENTS

INTRODUCTION

CHAPTER ONE

CHAPTER TWO

CHAPTER THREE

CHAPTER FOUR

CHAPTER NINE

CHAPTER TEN

EPILOGUE

INTRODUCTION

In a world where the allure of quick-fix diets and miracle weight loss solutions is hard to escape, there exists a distinct challenge for individuals living with diabetes who also seek to shed excess weight. This book, "Nourish and Slim: A Guide to Diabetic Weight Loss Through Balanced Nutrition," aims to break the barriers between sustainable weight loss and effective diabetes management, all while fostering a profound understanding of the pivotal role nutrition plays in this dual journey.

For millions, the diagnosis of diabetes can be a daunting prospect, laden with lifestyle adjustments and medical considerations. Yet, in the realm of weight loss, where confusion often clouds the path to wellness, individuals with diabetes face even greater complexity. Balancing the intricate dance between blood sugar regulation, nourishment, and weight loss requires more than a one-size-fits-all approach; it necessitates knowledge, empowerment, and the tools to navigate this intricate landscape.

"Nourish and Slim" is not just another diet book; it is an enlightening exploration of the symbiotic relationship between diabetes management and sustainable weight loss. Through the pages of this comprehensive guide, we will delve into the science behind diabetes, understanding the intricate interplay between insulin, blood sugar, and metabolism. With this foundational knowledge, we will then embark on an exciting journey to discover how thoughtful, balanced nutrition can be harnessed as a potent force in achieving both weight loss and optimal diabetes control.

This book is rooted in the principle that informed choices are the cornerstone of progress. Armed with the latest research, expert insights, and practical guidance, readers will be equipped to make mindful decisions about what they eat, when they eat, and how they can effectively manage their diabetes while shedding unwanted pounds. From crafting personalized meal plans to decoding food labels, from deciphering glycemic indices to exploring the psychology of eating, "Nourish and Slim" covers a breadth of topics designed to empower readers with the holistic understanding they need to rewrite their health narratives.

As we navigate the chapters ahead, we will debunk myths, unveil truths, and provide you with the tools you need to embrace a lifestyle that nourishes your body, minds, and aspirations. So, if you're ready to embark on a journey that merges the art and science of nutrition, diabetes management, and weight loss, turn the page and let us begin together on the path to wellness that's sustainable, sensible, and satisfying.

CHAPTER ONE

Understanding Diabetes and Weight Loss

1.1: The Intersection of Diabetes and Weight Management

Diabetes and weight management are intimately intertwined aspects of health, each influencing the other in complex ways. This section uncovers the dynamic relationship between diabetes and weight loss, highlighting how uncontrolled diabetes can impede weight loss efforts and vice versa. Readers will gain insight into how blood sugar levels, insulin resistance, and metabolism impact the body's ability to shed pounds effectively.

1.2: Types of Diabetes: Impact on Weight and Health

Delving deeper, this section provides a comprehensive overview of the different types of diabetes – type 1, type 2, and gestational diabetes – and their varying effects on weight and overall well-being. By understanding the unique characteristics of each type, readers will gain clarity on how diabetes diagnosis may influence weight loss strategies, offering a foundation for tailored approaches.

1.3: Unveiling the Science: Insulin, Blood Sugar, and Metabolism

In this scientifically grounded section, we delve into the intricate workings of insulin, blood sugar regulation, and metabolism. From insulin's role as a key regulator of glucose to the impact of insulin resistance on weight gain, readers will develop a clear comprehension of the physiological mechanisms underlying diabetes and weight management. This knowledge will empower readers to make informed choices and design strategies that work harmoniously with their bodies.

Through Section 1.1, 1.2, and 1.3, this chapter sets the stage for a comprehensive exploration of the intersection between diabetes and weight loss. By elucidating the underlying science and factors at play, readers will be better equipped to embark on a journey of balanced nutrition that takes into account their unique circumstances, ultimately paving the way for successful and sustainable diabetic weight management.

CHAPTER TWO

The Foundation of Balanced Nutrition

2.1: Building Blocks of a Diabetic-Friendly Diet

This section establishes the fundamental principles of crafting a diabetic-friendly diet. Readers will gain insight into the importance of nutrient-dense foods and discover the essential components that form the bedrock of their nutritional choices. Discussions on whole grains, lean proteins, healthy fats, and an array of fruits and vegetables will provide a comprehensive understanding of the building blocks necessary for optimal health and weight management.

2.2: The Role of Macronutrients in Diabetes and Weight Loss

Delving deeper, this section dissects the role of macronutrients – carbohydrates, proteins, and fats – in the context of diabetes and weight loss. Readers will explore how each macronutrient impacts blood sugar levels, energy expenditure, and overall metabolic function. By elucidating the benefits of balanced macronutrient consumption, readers will be equipped to create meals that not only satiate hunger but also contribute to stabilized blood sugar levels and effective weight loss.

2.3: Micronutrients: Small but Significant Contributors

This section shifts the focus to micronutrients – the vitamins, minerals, and antioxidants that play a vital role in supporting overall health and diabetes management. Readers will delve into the importance of micronutrients for immune function, cellular health, and metabolic processes. Additionally, the section highlights key micronutrients with specific benefits for individuals with diabetes, reinforcing the importance of a well-rounded, nutrient-rich diet. Through Section 2.1, 2.2, and 2.3, this chapter lays the groundwork for informed nutritional choices. By comprehending the significance of nutrient-dense foods, understanding the impact of macronutrients, and appreciating the role of micronutrients, readers will develop a comprehensive perspective on how their dietary decisions influence both their diabetes management and weight loss goals. Armed with this knowledge, they will be better equipped to embark on a journey of balanced nutrition and optimal well-being.

CHAPTER THREE

Crafting Your Diabetic Weight Loss Plan

3.1: Setting Realistic Goals for Success

In this section, readers will learn the art of goal setting, a crucial step towards achieving successful diabetic weight loss. By understanding the significance of specific, measurable, achievable, relevant, and time-bound (SMART) goals, readers will be equipped to define targets that are both attainable and motivating. Practical strategies for adapting goals to individual preferences and circumstances will also be explored.

3.2: Tailoring Your Plan to Your Body and Needs

This section delves into the importance of personalized approaches to diabetic weight loss. Readers will discover how factors such as age, activity level, medical history, and food preferences influence the design of an effective weight loss plan. Through actionable insights, readers will learn how to leverage their unique characteristics to tailor a plan that maximizes results and sustainability.

3.3: Meal Planning and Portion Control for Diabetes and Weight Management

Meal planning is a cornerstone of successful diabetic weight loss. In this section, readers will be guided through the process of creating balanced and nourishing meal plans. The concept of carbohydrate counting and its relevance to blood sugar management will be demystified, empowering readers to make informed choices about portion sizes and meal compositions. Practical tips for incorporating variety and flexibility into meal planning will also be provided.

Through Section 3.1, 3.2, and 3.3, this chapter equips readers with the tools to build a personalized and effective diabetic weight loss plan. By setting realistic goals, tailoring strategies to individual needs, and mastering meal planning and portion control, readers will gain the confidence to embark on a journey that is both empowering and sustainable. This chapter serves as a roadmap for transforming intentions into actionable steps and nurturing the path towards balanced nutrition, improved diabetes management, and successful weight loss.

CHAPTER FOUR

The Glycemic Index and Beyond

4.1: Demystifying the Glycemic Index

In this section, readers will delve into the concept of the glycemic index (GI) and its significance in diabetic weight loss. The chapter explains how different foods affect blood sugar levels and introduces readers to the GI scale. Through clear examples and practical explanations, readers will learn how to use the GI as a tool to make informed food choices that support stable blood sugar levels and effective weight management.

4.2: The Impact of Carbohydrates on Blood Sugar and Weight

This section expands on the role of carbohydrates in diabetes and weight loss. Readers will explore the intricate relationship between carbohydrates, blood sugar response, and insulin secretion. By gaining a deeper understanding of complex carbohydrates, simple sugars, and dietary fiber, readers will be empowered to make mindful carbohydrate choices that align with their health and weight loss goals.

4.3: Leveraging the Glycemic Load for Optimal Eating

Building on the foundation of the GI, this section introduces readers to the concept of glycemic load (GL), a dynamic approach to assessing the impact of carbohydrates on blood sugar levels. Readers will learn how to combine the GI and GL to make more accurate and nuanced food choices. Practical examples and strategies for selecting low-GI and low-

GL foods will be provided, offering readers the tools to create balanced and satisfying meals.

Through Section 4.1, 4.2, and 4.3, this chapter demystifies the intricacies of the glycemic index and empowers readers with the knowledge to navigate carbohydrate choices for improved diabetic weight loss. By understanding the impact of different carbohydrates on blood sugar levels and harnessing the power of the glycemic load, readers will be better equipped to create meals that support stable energy levels, effective weight management, and overall well-being. This chapter serves as a valuable resource for making informed dietary decisions that align with both diabetes management and weight loss goals.

CHAPTER FIVE

Mindful Eating and Psychological Well-being

5.1: Mind-Body Connection: Emotions and Eating Habits

In this section, readers will explore the intricate relationship between emotions and eating habits. By delving into the concept of emotional eating, readers will gain insight into how stress, boredom, and other emotional triggers can impact dietary choices. Practical exercises and strategies for cultivating self-awareness around emotional eating will be provided, empowering readers to develop a healthier relationship with food.

5.2: Strategies for Mindful Eating with Diabetes

Building on the foundation of emotional awareness, this section introduces the practice of mindful eating as a powerful tool for diabetes management and weight loss. Readers will learn how to engage their senses, savor each bite, and tune into hunger and fullness cues. Through guided mindfulness exercises and real-life examples, readers will discover how mindful eating can enhance their overall eating experience and support their health goals.

5.3: Overcoming Emotional Eating and Staying on Track

In this concluding section, readers will delve into actionable strategies for overcoming emotional eating patterns and maintaining consistency on their weight loss journey. From stress management techniques to building a supportive environment, readers will be equipped with practical tools to navigate challenges and setbacks. By understanding the role of psychological well-being in weight loss, readers will be better prepared to sustain positive habits and foster long-term success.

Through Section 5.1, 5.2, and 5.3, this chapter delves into the profound connection between the mind and eating habits. By cultivating emotional awareness, embracing mindful eating, and developing strategies for psychological well-being, readers will be empowered to make conscious, healthful choices that not only support diabetes management but also contribute to effective weight loss. This chapter serves as a comprehensive guide for nourishing both body and mind, fostering a harmonious and sustainable approach to achieving health and wellness goals.

CHAPTER SIX

Navigating the Supermarket and Beyond

6.1: Decoding Food Labels: Hidden Sugars and More

In this section, readers will embark on a journey through the aisles of the supermarket, equipped with the knowledge to decipher food labels effectively. By understanding the various names for added sugars, recognizing common culprits, and identifying other key nutritional information, readers will gain the skills to make informed choices that align with their diabetic weight loss goals.

6.2: Smart Grocery Shopping for Diabetic Weight Loss

Building on label reading, this section guides readers in creating a strategic grocery shopping plan that supports their dietary objectives. From compiling a well-rounded shopping list to navigating different sections of the store, readers will learn how to stock their kitchen with nutrient-rich, diabetes-friendly foods. Practical tips for avoiding impulse purchases and optimizing grocery trips will also be explored.

6.3: Dining Out and Traveling: Making Healthy Choices Everywhere

In this final section, readers will discover strategies for maintaining their diabetic weight loss plan in situations that extend beyond the supermarket. From dining out at restaurants to navigating travel and social gatherings, readers will be equipped with tools to make mindful choices, communicate dietary needs effectively, and adapt their eating habits to various settings. Practical guidance for prioritizing health while enjoying life's experiences will be provided.

Through Section 6.1, 6.2, and 6.3, this chapter empowers readers with the skills to navigate food choices beyond their kitchen. By decoding food labels, optimizing grocery shopping, and mastering dining out and travel scenarios, readers will be prepared to make health-conscious decisions that align with their diabetic weight loss journey. This chapter serves as a comprehensive guide to extending healthy habits beyond the home, ensuring that readers can continue making progress towards their goals no matter where life takes them.

CHAPTER SEVEN

Cooking and Creating Diabetic-Friendly Delights

7.1: From the Kitchen to the Table: Culinary Techniques for Health

In this section, readers will embark on a culinary exploration, learning how to transform fresh ingredients into flavorful, diabetes-friendly meals. Through discussions on cooking methods, seasoning alternatives, and healthier preparation techniques, readers will gain the skills to create delicious dishes that support their weight loss and diabetes management goals.

7.2: Flavor without Compromise: Recipes for Diabetic Weight Loss

Building upon culinary techniques, this section provides a curated selection of diabetic-friendly recipes. Readers will explore a diverse array of dishes, from breakfast options to satisfying dinners and delightful desserts. Each recipe is thoughtfully crafted to balance taste and nutrition, incorporating whole foods and mindful ingredient substitutions to promote satiety and stable blood sugar levels.

7.3: Meal Prep and Batch Cooking for Convenience and Success

In this concluding section, readers will discover the art of meal prep and batch cooking as strategies for maintaining consistency and efficiency in their diabetic weight loss journey. Practical tips for planning meals ahead, storing prepared ingredients, and assembling balanced meals on busy days will be shared. By mastering the art of preparation, readers can navigate their daily routines with ease, ensuring that nutritious options are always within reach.

Through Section 7.1, 7.2, and 7.3, this chapter elevates readers' culinary skills and empowers them to take charge of their dietary choices. By learning cooking techniques, exploring flavorful recipes, and embracing meal prep strategies, readers will not only enhance their ability to create delicious and nourishing meals but also solidify their commitment to sustainable diabetic weight loss. This chapter serves as a comprehensive guide to embracing the joy of cooking and celebrating the synergy of taste and health.

CHAPTER EIGHT

Exercise, Movement, and Metabolism Boosting

8.1: Exercise's Impact on Diabetes Management and Weight Loss

This section introduces readers to the powerful role that exercise plays in diabetes management and weight loss. Readers will explore the physiological benefits of physical activity, including improved insulin sensitivity, enhanced metabolism, and increased energy expenditure. Practical insights into how exercise influences blood sugar levels and supports overall health will provide a foundation for the chapters to come.

8.2: Finding the Right Workouts for Your Body and Lifestyle

Building on the understanding of exercise's impact, this section guides readers in selecting appropriate workouts tailored to their individual needs and preferences. Readers will explore various types of exercises – from aerobic to strength training, flexibility to high-intensity interval training (HIIT) – and discover how to create a well-rounded exercise routine that not only promotes weight loss but also contributes to overall fitness and well-being.

8.3: Staying Active: Incorporating Movement Throughout Your Day

In this concluding section, readers will learn practical strategies for integrating movement seamlessly into their daily lives. The concept of non-exercise activity thermogenesis (NEAT) will be explored, emphasizing the importance of small, consistent movements in supporting weight loss and metabolic health. Readers will discover tips for staying active at home, work, and during leisure activities, ensuring that movement becomes a natural and integral part of their routine.

Through Section 8.1, 8.2, and 8.3, this chapter empowers readers to harness the benefits of exercise for diabetes management and weight loss. By understanding exercise's impact on the body, tailoring workouts to individual preferences, and embracing a lifestyle of consistent movement, readers will be equipped to create a comprehensive approach to health that goes beyond the plate. This chapter serves as a dynamic guide to embracing physical activity as a key component of the journey towards improved well-being and sustainable weight loss.

CHAPTER NINE

Support, Sustainability, and Long-Term Success

9.1: The Importance of Support Networks and Accountability

In this section, readers will discover the significance of building a strong support network to facilitate their diabetic weight loss journey. The chapter explores the role of friends, family, and healthcare professionals in providing encouragement, guidance, and accountability. Readers will also learn practical strategies for communicating their goals and needs, fostering an environment that fosters success.

9.2: Overcoming Plateaus and Challenges Along the Way

Building upon the concept of support, this section equips readers with strategies to overcome common challenges and plateaus that may arise during their journey. From addressing weight loss plateaus to managing stressors and setbacks, readers will learn how to navigate obstacles with resilience and adaptability. Practical advice for problem-solving and staying motivated will empower readers to continue making progress despite hurdles.

9.3: Cultivating a Lifestyle that Sustains Diabetic Weight Loss

In this concluding section, readers will explore the art of transitioning from a weight loss-focused approach to a sustainable, lifelong lifestyle that supports diabetes management and overall well-being. Readers will learn how to integrate the principles they've acquired throughout the book into their daily routines, ensuring that healthy habits become second nature. The section provides guidance on setting new goals, maintaining progress, and celebrating achievements as part of an ongoing journey towards optimal health.

Through Section 9.1, 9.2, and 9.3, this chapter lays the groundwork for readers to achieve long-term success in their diabetic weight loss endeavors. By understanding the importance of support, mastering strategies for overcoming challenges, and embracing a sustainable lifestyle, readers will be equipped with the tools to navigate their ongoing journey with confidence and purpose. This chapter serves as a comprehensive guide to fostering resilience, maintaining progress, and cultivating a balanced, health-focused approach that extends far beyond the confines of weight loss goals.

CHAPTER TEN

Your Journey Ahead: Embracing Wellness

10.1: Celebrating Milestones and Non-Scale Victories

In this section, readers will learn the art of celebrating progress beyond just numbers on a scale. The chapter highlights the importance of acknowledging and appreciating non-scale victories – such as improved energy levels, better blood sugar control, and increased mobility. Readers will discover how these victories contribute to a sense of accomplishment and motivate continued commitment to their diabetic weight loss journey.

10.2: Navigating Setbacks: Turning Challenges into Opportunities

Building upon the concept of celebrating milestones, this section equips readers with a resilient mindset to navigate setbacks and challenges. Readers will learn how to reframe setbacks as learning experiences, using them as opportunities to refine strategies and enhance their approach to diabetes management and weight loss. Practical tools for managing setbacks and maintaining a positive outlook will empower readers to overcome obstacles with grace and determination.

10.3: Looking Forward: A Future of Health, Balance, and Vitality

In this concluding section, readers will be guided to envision their future through a lens of health, balance, and vitality. The chapter explores the transformative potential of embracing a holistic approach to well-being, where diabetic weight loss is one facet of a multi-faceted lifestyle. Readers will discover how the principles and knowledge acquired throughout the book can shape a future that encompasses physical, emotional, and mental well-being.

Through Section 10.1, 10.2, and 10.3, this chapter serves as a bridge between the present and the future, guiding readers towards a life enriched by health and vitality. By celebrating milestones, adopting a resilient mindset, and looking forward to a future of holistic well-being, readers will be inspired to continue their journey with a sense of purpose and optimism. This chapter encapsulates the essence of the book's message, inviting readers to embrace wellness as a lifelong pursuit that extends far beyond the final page.

EPILOGUE

Embracing Your Journey to Wellness

As we come to the close of "Nourish and Slim: A Guide to Diabetic Weight Loss Through Balanced Nutrition," we reflect upon the enlightening voyage we've embarked upon. Throughout these pages, we've navigated the intricate pathways of diabetes management, weight loss, and the profound connection between the two. From understanding the interplay of insulin and metabolism to crafting nutritious meals that nourish body and soul, we've delved deep into the art and science of balanced nutrition.

In our journey together, we've explored not just the "what" but also the "why" and "how" behind diabetic weight loss. We've embraced the power of goal setting, tailored strategies, and the impact of mindfulness on our dietary choices. We've decoded food labels, mastered the art of preparation, and discovered the myriad ways to incorporate movement into our daily lives. We've learned to face challenges with resilience, celebrating victories large and small, and fostering a mindset that turns setbacks into stepping stones toward progress.

As we turn our gaze towards the horizon, the epilogue invites you to take a moment of reflection. You've not only gained knowledge but also embarked on a transformative journey that transcends the confines of these pages. The principles, strategies, and insights you've acquired are not merely tools for today but guiding lights for the future.

Your journey towards wellness is a testament to your commitment, your courage, and your dedication to a life that embodies health, balance, and vitality. The path ahead may hold its twists and turns, but armed with the knowledge and wisdom gained from this book, you have the power to navigate with confidence, purpose, and grace.

In this epilogue, we celebrate your journey thus far and invite you to continue embracing wellness in all its dimensions. The culmination of your efforts is not an ending but a new beginning, a chapter in a story that is uniquely yours. May you walk this path with a heart full of hope, a mind attuned to possibilities, and a spirit ever eager to embrace the richness of a life well-lived.

As the pages of this book come to a close, remember that your journey towards wellness is a lifelong endeavor – an ongoing narrative of growth, self-discovery, and transformation. Your story continues beyond these words, and we wish you nothing but the very best as you step forward into a future brimming with health, balance, and vitality.

With gratitude and inspiration,

Williams Acheson